THE
HEMP
MANIFESTO

THE
HEMP
MANIFESTO

101
Ways That
Hemp Can
Save Our
World

ROWAN ROBINSON

Park Street Press
Rochester, Vermont

Park Street Press
One Park Street
Rochester, Vermont 05767
www.gotoit.com

Library of Congress Cataloging-in-Publication Data
Robinson, Rowan.
   The hemp manifesto : 101 ways that hemp can save our world / Rowan Robinson
       p.   cm.
   ISBN 978-089281728-3
   1. Hemp—Miscellanea.   2. Cannabis—Miscellanea.   I. Title.
SB255.R635   1997
677'.12—dc21   97-20759
                                              CIP

Printed and bound in India

10 9 8 7 6 5 4

Text design and layout by Kristin Camp
This book was typeset in Stone Sans with Greco Deco as the
   display typeface

Park Street Press is a division of Inner Traditions International

Though I do not believe that a plant will spring up where no seed has been, I have great faith in a seed. Convince me that you have a seed there, and I am prepared to expect wonders.

Henry David Thoreau

INTRODUCTION

Chances are if you've picked up this book, you already know a bit about hemp. Maybe you've read about hemp's potential to replace trees as the source of paper, and cotton as the source of textiles. Maybe you've even bought yourself a hemp wallet or vest. Or perhaps you are one of the growing number of people who has discovered the delicious taste of hempseed foods.

On the other hand, you may be one of the people in Arizona or California who helped pass the propositions legalizing hemp's therapeutic cousin, medical marijuana, in the 1996 elections. You may even have cancer or AIDS yourself, and know firsthand the healing properties of the plant.

Then again, maybe you've never seen a hemp product or a marijuana cigarette in your life, but you are a firm believer in the democratic process and have an abiding interest in the environmental, economic, and physical health of your country and its people.

Whatever the case, you've undoubtedly had an experience similar to this: when you tell people some of the incredible facts you've learned, they are skeptical, amazed that a plant they've always been told was a national scourge has actually proved so useful to so many for so long. But if you tell them enough, they become fascinated and want to know more—or at least want proof.

Here's where you run into problems. They aren't ready to drop twenty dollars on a book about hemp, and they certainly aren't going to wait around while you flip through pages hunting for confirmation of what you've been saying. This is when you pull your *Hemp Manifesto* out of your back pocket and press it into their palm. The facts are all here, easy to find and incontrovertible; guaranteed to make even the most skeptical listener curious enough to want to know more.

And that is the key. Education is the only way to overcome ignorance, and ignorance is the only thing holding the hemp revolution back. Because once people have the facts, they see what a good thing this plant is. This particularly applies to law enforcement and legislative bodies, both of which have been shockingly thick-headed on this issue. They are not about to educate the public on the history and current uses of cannabis, and have even worked to *prevent* the public from learning the facts. Though a reversal of policy on cannabis would benefit government greatly in the long run, it would be inconvenient in the short run and require some real thinking, and this is not something government does easily.

Hence, as with all revolutions, this one must begin with the people and work its way up. Once government sees how out of step with the people it has become, it will be forced to change. The pressure has already begun; it is my sincere hope that *The Hemp Manifesto* will help tighten the vise a few more turns.

There are two separate issues in *The Hemp Manifesto,* and their confusion has caused many a problem for the hemp movement, so it is important to clarify them here. Both hemp and marijuana are members of the same species, *Cannabis sativa.* This does not make them the same plant. Think of a beagle and a Saint Bernard—both *Canis familiaris,* but with utterly different looks, capabilities, and personalities. So it is with hemp and marijuana.

Hemp is a stalky crop that has been grown for its fiber and edible seed for millennia; it is incapable of getting you stoned. Marijuana is a bushy form of cannabis that has been grown for its psycho-active and medicinal properties for an equally long time. The two are different plants and in two minutes a state trooper can be educated so that he will never mistake one for the other.

To avoid confusion, the first part of this book concentrates on ways that nonpsychoactive hemp has made, is making, or could make a positive impact on the world. The second part then concentrates on marijuana. The two are separate issues and you can be legitimately and completely in favor of one and against the other. But one of the truly remarkable things about *Cannabis sativa* is that one form of it has served humanity in the most utilitarian ways, while the other has appealed to our most spiritual and cerebral nature. Thus it seems entirely appropriate to celebrate the dual nature of this age-old ally in one book.

SAVING THE FOREST

The industrial world's hunger for wood has already destroyed 97 percent of the mature forests of North America and the rest of the world's forests are following close behind. Not only are forests the key to preventing loss of topsoil and pollution of waterways, they are also home to most of the world's terrestrial species and the source of much of the world's oxygen.

Half the trees cut down are used to make paper products, yet hemp could provide for all our paper needs. An acre of hemp yields four times as much fiber as an acre of trees, and no wildlife is destroyed in the process. With hemp we can feed our paper industry and let the forests regenerate at the same time.

PAPER FOR
THE LONG HAUL

Hemp was the world's first source of paper, invented in China around 100 B.C. Two-thousand-year-old pieces of hemp paper have stood the test of time, a feat far beyond the capabilities of wood pulp paper. In fact, if wood pulp had been the source of paper throughout history, it is terrifying to think of the history and literature we would know nothing about, for—until the development of acid-free paper—wood pulp paper disintegrated after little more than a century. A return to hemp paper would make the acid-free paper process unnecessary. Hemp paper is also stronger than wood pulp paper, naturally pliable, and partially water-resistant.

FIBERBOARD

Fiberboard—composite board made from processed wood chips and resins—is used in cabinetry, paneling, furniture, and any other place where nonstructural wood is needed. It is one of the fastest growing segments of the wood industry. But fiberboard made from wood chips is notoriously weak. Hemp, with its long bast fibers, makes far stronger fiberboard, and thus has a wider range of applications. It is also more fireproof and insect-resistant.

INSULATION

Just as hemp fiber can replace fiberglass in cars, boats, skateboards, and other solid fiberglass products, it also makes a perfect substitute for that other famous fiberglass material: insulation. Hemp hurds (the inner core of the hemp stalk, high in cellulose) are treated with a fire retardant and then blown into space between walls. Hemp insulation produces neither the lung nor skin irritation associated with fiberglass insulation.

A MAN'S HEMP
IS HIS CASTLE

Isochanvre, a French company, has patented a concrete substitute made by calcifying hemp stalks into a solid mass. The resulting material, also known as isochanvre, is as strong as concrete but weighs only one-seventh as much. In addition, it is more flexible, thus better able to withstand natural disasters, and is a much better insulator.

The company has already built hundreds of these all-natural houses in Europe, and the first has appeared in Canada as well. A commitment to these efficient, economical houses would significantly lessen the impact of drilling and mining on the environment.

SHOWER CURTAINS

Shower curtains are just one of the many plastic products that release toxic gasses when heated. Unfortunately, shower curtains tend to be heated a lot. Rather than be trapped in a small confined space and gassed by your shower curtain, switch to Hungarian hemp shower curtains, now on the market. Attractive, long-lasting, and naturally mildew resistant, they are the healthy alternative for your immediate environment as well as your global one.

NATURAL HERBICIDE

Herbicides are bad news, we know. They keep weeds down, but they poison the ground with unnatural chemicals that make our food supply, our selves, and our world sick.

Hemp has been used for centuries as a natural herbicide, in places as diverse as Kentucky and Siberia. Capable of growing six feet in two weeks, the thickly sowed hemp crop simply outcompetes all weeds in sight, choking them off from sunlight and nutrients. So successful is hemp at doing this that it sometimes has been grown purely for this purpose. But why limit yourself? Hemp rotated with another crop leaves your soil in prime shape for whatever follows and gives you an extra cash crop for your trouble. All without ever touching a chemical of any kind.

THE MUDDY GANGES

Massive deforestation on the slopes of the Himalayas—hemp's original home—is quickly turning that cradle of spirituality into a barren moonscape. Forested areas that previously lost only .03 tons of soil per hectare each year lose as much as 90 tons per hectare after being clearcut. At that rate soon nothing but rock is left. The soil washes downstream, clogging rivers and killing acquatic life, and eventually is swept into the sea by the Ganges and other rivers. Vice President Al Gore himself says, "These mountain lands, which boast some of the most spectacular natural beauty on earth, are now being devastated to briefly quench the needs of a single generation."

Hemp, which grows abundantly in the Himalayas when given a chance, can cover these scarred areas with a green bandage of roots, stalks, and leaves that will hold the soil in place and provide an income for the region's people.

THE FABRIC
OF HEALTHY LIVES

Not cotton. Cotton is one of the most destructive crops in existence. Half the pesticides used in the United States go to cotton alone, which is grown on 3 percent of the world's best arable land but is responsible for 26 percent of the pesticides. Even organic cotton requires extremely heavy irrigation, which ruins the water table and encourages erosion. Continued use of cotton is the best way to ensure that a second Dust Bowl will occur.

Hemp, which can be grown organically and sustainably, can be used to make all the textiles we currently make from cotton. Indeed, hemp was our primary source of clothing for centuries until the cotton gin made harvesting of cotton extremely inexpensive. In 1776 a hemp shirt cost $1 while a cotton shirt cost $100. With minor alterations, our entire textile industry could switch to hemp, significantly reducing the amount of chemicals that soak into our soil and waterways.

THE FABRIC
OF STYLING LIVES

Hemp makes extremely attractive clothing. Its long bast fibers can be spun into fabric that is stronger and thinner than cotton, similar to linen or raw silk. The natural, relaxed hang of hemp is a look that is contemporary and classic at the same time, and is already becoming a symbol for those who have a progressive view of the world's future.

CLEAN HEMPAHOL

Corn is not the only plant that can be used to make ethanol. The carbohydrate molecules in almost any agricultural crop can be broken down into a fuel source just as efficient as the gasoline derived from the hydrocarbon molecules in fossil fuels. Per acre, hemp is a more prolific producer of ethanol than corn.

Unlike gasoline, ethanol does not produce any of the sulfur or other air pollution responsible for acid rain and various diseases. Conversion of automobile engines from gas-burning to ethanol-burning would dramatically clean the world's air.

NO OIL SPILLS

The point is so obvious that it might easily be missed, and is worth stating: hemp causes no oil spills. A world that relies on locally produced hemp ethanol rather than imported oil is a world that never has to see scenes such as the one left by the Exxon *Valdez:* hundreds of miles of pristine coastline and thousands of birds and marine animals choked to death by black oil slicks. A world without oil slicks is a beautiful thing.

NO GULF WAR

If the world relied on energy crops like hemp instead of oil the Gulf War never would have happened. No more would countries desperate for oil battle each other over desert land. Agricultural crops are *renewable* sources of energy, and can be grown in virtually every country on earth. They would free much of the world's people from reliance on more powerful or more fortunate nations for their energy needs. Unless a change to agricultural biomass energy is begun soon, as the world's oil supplies run dry the oil wars will only get more brutal.

BOTTOMS UP!

Don't forget to count your baby among the new breed of hempsters. Hemp makes the best diapers in the world. Reusable, it doesn't fill landfills, as plastic diapers do. And hemp is far more absorbent than cotton, making baby and parents alike drier than do cotton diapers.

SUSTAINABILITY

Any natural resource we use that is not getting re-supplied at an equal rate will eventually leave us empty-handed. Think of your bank account. It generates interest, and if you spend only the interest each month, or if you deposit as much as you withdraw, then you can sustain yourself indefinitely. If you consistently spend the capital, however, eventually the bill comes due and you're bankrupt.

Right now the human race is blowing its wad with mind-boggling speed. Our bank account was started by Mother Earth long ago and consists of soil, forests, fossil fuels, and other materials. It generates a little interest all by itself each year, but we are burning up all the interest and a great deal of the capital, and the bill is on its way to the table.

Using hemp for our material needs can be done on a *sustainable* basis, a balanced cycle of matter and energy. It isn't really a question of choice; it's just a matter of time.

A WIN-WIN SITUATION

A nasty side effect of many factories and mining operations is that the surrounding soil gets saturated with concentrations of heavy metals, turning it toxic for centuries. Hemp has been demonstrated to draw heavy metals up through its roots, storing them in its stalk. That's right: several seasons of hemp can literally *clean* polluted soil. The stalks can then be used for fiberboard, paper, insulation, plastic polymers; any use where they aren't combusted.

AIRING OUT
THE GREENHOUSE

Everyone is now familiar with the greenhouse effect, where carbon dioxide released from burning fuels and breathing animals acts like the panes of glass in a greenhouse, preventing heat from escaping the earth and dangerously raising the planet's temperature.

Replacing fossil fuels with hemp as our primary energy source mitigates the greenhouse effect. Growing hemp cycles carbon dioxide out of the air and replaces it with oxygen, restoring the planet's atmosphere to its natural balance.

STRONGER RECYCLED PAPER

Many paper recyclers around the world have to buy wastepaper from suppliers because local recycling efforts are not large enough to meet their demands. Hemp, grown locally, could supplement the regional supply, bringing wages to locals and eliminating the need for importing wastepaper. Hemp's long fibers also increase the durability of recycled paper, which weakens with each cycle of use.

THE HEMPMOBILE

In the 1930s the great American innovator Henry Ford foresaw a future in which we would no longer have to mine the earth, polluting air and groundwater for centuries, in order to get metal to build our automobiles. Plastic was the future. Only problem? Plastic was made from oil, and oil meant reliance on foreign powers. But there was a secret the oil industry did not want anyone to know: anything made from the hydrocarbons in oil could just as easily be made from the carbohydrates in vegetable crops. Henry did just this, making a car "grown from the soil" out of hemp and other annual crops. The car was considerably more durable than its steel counterpart thanks to the hemp fiber in it.

What goes around comes around, and today the German auto manufacturer Daimler-Benz is experimenting with a hempmobile of its own. The advantage? It is all-organic and completely recyclable.

THE QUEEN'S STEED

Hemp is the most prized material for animal bedding in the world. The high percentage of cellulose in its stalk makes it extremely absorbent. It has been used in Europe for this purpose for centuries. Much of the hemp currently grown in England goes to this purpose, and the queen herself provides her horse with a bed of hemp and nothing but.

GRASSGLASS

The fiber in fiberglass is easily replaced with hemp fiber, making a durable, naturally grown product that you could call *grassglass*. Besides insulation, grassglass is ideal for skateboards, boats, even automobile interiors. Several automotive companies are currently experimenting with its use.

SNOWBOARDS

You aren't cool on the slopes anymore unless you're riding on hemp. That's ever since Marvin Christianson's company Bigfoot came up with their hemp snowboard. Consisting of a wood core wrapped with hemp fabric and decorated with hemp twill, the board is light, durable, and environmentally friendly. And, most importantly if you're a snowboarder, it's on the cutting edge of hip.

THE PEOPLE
V.
WOODY HARRELSON

On June 1, 1996, the actor Woody Harrelson was arrested for planting four seeds of industrial hemp in Beattyville, Kentucky. The previous day Harrelson had held a press conference on hemp and announced an essay contest for grade schoolers in Kentucky. After his arrest, Harrelson said, "I planted industrial hemp and got arrested because someone must highlight this difference, and in order to truly know the law one must test the law. I think it is time for all of us to make a stand."

Thus Harrelson became the latest in a long line of great Americans who have used civil disobedience as a means of saving a part of the world despite empty laws. On January 23, 1997, a judge ruled that not differentiating between hemp and marijuana is unconstitutional.

BALANCE OF POWER

The United States may turn its nose up at the prospect of a hemp industry, but other less fortunate nations know a good thing when they see it. The leading producers of hemp are nations such as Ukraine, China, Romania, and Hungary. It is rare for these nations to be out in front of the Western world in any industry, and this one is no coincidence. In all these nations hemp is a traditional part of the culture. They continued growing it when it was long forgotten in more advanced nations, and, for now at least, they are reaping the rewards. It will be years before the United States can catch up with them.

FARM-AID

All over the United States, farmland is lying fallow when it could be growing hemp. Hemp makes an excellent rotation crop with corn, enabling a farmer to get more than twice the profits out of the same soil while keeping it free of weeds for the next crop. This caused singer Willie Nelson to say that hemp "could make the very difference between the survival of the family farm and its extinction. It is much more valuable than corn or other grains and has many markets."

The American Farm Bureau, the largest farming organization in the United States and one hardly known for its radical stances, is so enthusiastic about hemp's potential that it passed a unanimous resolution in 1996 to "encourage research into the viability and economic potential of industrial hemp production."

NATIVE HEMP

The confusion of the U.S. government regarding industrial hemp may turn into a windfall for the country's original occupants. Native American tribes, including the Navajo, Tuskarora, and Oglala Sioux, are all investigating growing hemp on tribal lands. These lands are not under the jurisdiction of the federal government. Having a monopoly on the domestic hemp crop could give these tribes an excellent and stable economic base.

The Navajo Nation planted their initial hemp crop on March 17, 1996. Money to buy the seeds was raised by weaving and selling elaborate hemp tapestries. They eventually plan to grow 30,000 acres. In their official resolution they stated that their reason for growing hemp is to insure the future of Mother Earth.

TOBACCO SALVATION

Amid lawsuits, scandals, and an increasing non-smoking public, the tobacco industry is losing favor. This is good news, but the loss of thousands of jobs on farms and factories is not. Fortunately, salvation is at hand. Hemp can be grown in the same fields that now grow tobacco, and processed in many of the same factories that now produce cigarettes. This keeps everyone at work making a product that supports a sustainable future, rather than one that exhausts the soil, kills hundreds of thousands of people each year, and transfers immense health-care costs to each of us.

Don't take my word for it, take Thomas Jefferson's: "The best hemp and the best tobacco grow on the same kind of soil. The former article is of the first necessity to the . . . wealth and protection of the country. The latter, never useful and sometimes pernicious, derives its estimation from caprice. . . . Hemp becomes the means of support to numbers of people, hence it is to be preferred."

GO, CANADA

While the United States invents reasons why it cannot allow industrial hemp to be grown, Canada has no such qualms and government-sanctioned hemp crops have been growing there since 1995. Canada, which generally cannot compete economically with its southern neighbor, is way out in front on this one, and just may steal a badly needed industry for itself.

THIRD WORLD RELIEF

Hemp grows well in many areas of the world suffering from malnutrition and impoverishment, such as Africa. By encouraging large-scale hemp agriculture, organizations such as the Peace Corp can give African farmers a fiber crop that could be sold for good prices on the international market, significantly raising their standard of living. At the same time, the seed would provide farmers and their families with a high-quality source of food.

GRASSROOTS INDUSTRY

Until recently hemp was too controversial for any large companies that need to worry about public relations, so hemp became the province of young, idealistic entrepreneurs. These enterprising upstarts wanted to make money, sure, but they were in it to do some good, too. They were interested in hemp because of its environmental benefits, and were rewarded with an industry where they could make a living and make a small difference at the same time.

Today, though a few big-name companies such as Calvin Klein, Adidas, and Levis have dipped their toes into hempen waters, hemp is still a cottage industry. It is one of the few industries left where you can know that your money is finding its way into the hands of people who want to do their part to save the world.

ENLIGHTENED KIDS

Hemp is helping teach kids the difference between good deeds and self-serving government. Actor Woody Harrelson sponsors a contest for the best essays on the uses of industrial hemp by students in grades 4 to 12. Awards are given in three age categories. Harrelson said that kids "seem to understand [the issue] a lot better than adults. It seems very simple to them, and they didn't seem to confuse hemp with marijuana."

Teaching children to think for themselves and get their own information on a subject, rather than simply swallowing the official story, is one of the healthiest acts of a democratic society. Industrial hemp is a perfect lesson in the reality of American government.

BALANCING
THE IMBALANCE

The story of the 1990s has been the flight of manufacturing jobs out of the United States to cheaper foreign labor markets. Hemp is helping to make up for this loss of jobs. The majority of hemp products—from cosmetics to paper, textiles, and foods—are made in the United States, using imported hemp, by artisans and entrepreneurs who are making a living doing so. Hemp customers also place a healthy emphasis on quality, sustainability, and handmade touches that help support this anti-factory approach.

MOTHER OF MASTERPIECES

Hemp was the canvas on which many of the world's greatest oil paintings were created, including those of Rembrandt and Van Gogh. The Spanish artist Joan Miro's great tapestry that hangs in the World Trade Center is composed of wool and hemp.

IT'S PATRIOTIC (1)

When the fledgling republic cast around for a flag to embody its new spirit of independence, Betsy Ross was there with her needle and her hemp. Were it not for hemp, she might have had to paint the Stars and Stripes onto a deer hide. Somehow, a ragtag army of farmers waving deerskins over their heads would have been less inspiring, and the country might never have been the same.

IT'S PATRIOTIC (2)

Both the Declaration of Independence and the Constitution of the United States of America were drafted on hemp paper. George Washington, Thomas Jefferson, James Madison, John Adams, and America's other patriotic greats proudly put their names to hemp paper as no modern politician would dare to do. Washington and Jefferson grew acres of hemp, an activity that today would land them in jail for life.

HEMP FOR VICTORY!

Though hemp was banned in 1937, the United States suddenly reversed its position in 1942, *subsidized* the cultivation of the crop, and even made a short film urging farmers to grow it! What had changed? World War II.

Since 1937 the United States had been importing its hemp from the Far East. But with that supply cut off by the Japanese, the U.S. found itself in a bind. Every Navy battleship required 34,000 feet of hemp rope to keep running. Without hemp millions of GIs couldn't tie their shoes, and parachutes had no webbing. So hemp metamorphosed overnight from the evil weed to the patriotic crop. Hundreds of thousands of acres were grown under government contract to save the country. After the war the government flip-flopped once more, and hemp became the evil weed again. But who knows when it will be called upon next to save a person, country, or planet?

GETTING THE WORD OUT

And I do mean "the Word." When Johannes Gutenberg perfected movable type in the fifteenth century, he would have had nothing to print on without hemp. Hemp was responsible for almost all of the world's paper at that point, thus Gutenberg's famous Bible and most other books owed their existence to hemp. With the production of the printing press and a ready source of paper, literacy flourished in Europe and the Dark Ages were left behind in earnest.

THE SCYTHE

The Scythians were a fierce nomadic people from the Russian Steppes who swept into Europe around 700 B.C. They brought with them their hemp culture—they made clothing from its fiber and used its psychoactive properties in religious rites. They had developed a curved cutting tool perfect for harvesting the stalky plant, a tool superior to any used in Europe at that time. The tool helped revolutionize agriculture in Europe, and today still bears the name of the civilization that introduced it.

THE POWER OF CANVAS

One of the great leaps in human creativity was the invention of the sail. Wind power turned the seas from unconquerable monsters into ideal trade routes, and the first great age of exploration and commerce was on. The Arabs were the first people to master the triangular sail, and they also gave us the word for what that sail was made of—*canvas,* which they called *canefas,* from the Greek *kannabis.* Hemp, in other words. Hemp triggered the discovery of the New World, the establishment of worldwide trade routes, indeed the entire notion that the earth was primarily water with small islands of land, rather than land with occasional small seas in it. And the world has never looked back.

NATIONAL INDEPENDENCE

Thomas Jefferson believed hemp to be so important to the independence of the colonies that he secretly brought new varieties of it back from France, thus becoming the first cannabis smuggler on record. The profusion of hemp in the colonies provided an independent source of paper, clothing, rope, food, oil, and sails, and was one of the arguments Thomas Paine used in *Common Sense* to convince the colonists that they could secede from England.

Today, a healthy hemp industry still gives a nation economic independence by providing a source for all the basic needs of society, without reliance on foreign trade.

THE TEMPLES OF MAN

Ever wonder how the Egyptians moved the giant limestone blocks they used to build the pyramids? Only one substance was strong enough to allow hundreds of slaves to drag the blocks—hemp. Hemp cordage 4,000 years old has been found at Thebes. And bas-relief carvings show piles of hemp stalks being used for fiber while the tops of the plants are being crushed into incense—another favorite of the Egyptians, who considered cannabis incense to be particularly pleasing to the gods. Thus hemp made possible the construction of these holy places and enhanced the feelings of worship that inspired them.

PURITY

Contrary to the United States, in Japan hemp is considered such a superior plant that it has long been associated with purity itself. For this reason, hemp was the fabric of choice for religious ceremonial garb. The plant was considered so powerful a blessing that it was even used to drive away evil spirits. Shinto priests would attach undyed hemp fibers to one end of a stick and wave the stick over the heads of individuals thought to be possessed by spirits. Since it was believed that evil and purity could not coexist, the presence of the hemp would drive the evil away.

Hemp became the primary source of fabric for kimonos, and the naturally beautiful material allowed Japanese artisans to achieve unparalleled heights of craftsmanship.

SOY SHMOY!

Tired of tofu? Eaten enough soyburgers for one lifetime? Then you'll be glad to know that there's a better source of protein out there—you guessed it, hemp. The seeds of the hemp plant—actually classified as fruit—have served as a primary food source in China, India, and Russia for thousands of years. Each hemp plant can produce about a liter of seed, and about 25 percent of the seed is protein. This protein is the most complete protein to be found in the vegetable kingdom, and is more easily digested than soy protein and just as versatile.

And how does it taste? Nutty and delicious, most people say. But find out for yourself. Hempseed products are available throughout the United States and Europe, from SeedySweety snack bars to Hemprella cheese, Hempeh burgers, Cajun roasted hempseed, pure hempseed oil, hempseed flour, even hempseed oil ice cream! And the seed of the hemp plant is always THC-free, even seed obtained from psychoactive varieties.

EFAS—FOR SMART EATERS

Essential fatty acids (EFAs) are more important to the body than vitamins, yet they get far less attention. Fatty acids provide the lipids that keep cells fluid and flexible. While some of these can be manufactured by the body, essential fatty acids cannot and must be consumed in food. Hempseed oil is an excellent source of EFAs.

By keeping cells naturally flexible, EFAs help to regulate all processes within the body—especially the brain, which is composed largely of EFAs. Experiments with animals have shown that a diet deficient in EFAs can result in poor brain development, faulty immune function, dried tear ducts and salivary glands, slow-healing wounds, cardiovascular abnormalities, susceptibility to arthritis and inflammatory disorders, nonelastic skin, and poor reproduction. Thus hempseed should be considered an *essential* food source, especially for children, pregnant women, and nursing mothers.

OMEGA-3

In recent years scientists have discovered the powerful health benefits of one particular EFA—omega-3 fatty acid, found in cold-water oily fishes such as salmon, mackerel, and herring. This essential fatty acid has been proved to lower cholesterol levels and blood pressure, and to inhibit platelet coagulation—hardening of the arteries.

There are very few sources of omega-3 oil other than fish. The two best terrestrial sources are flaxseed oil and hempseed oil, but there is a major difference between the two. Hempseed oil has a wonderful natural flavor and makes excellent salad dressings, while flaxseed oil is known to make people gag and can cause skin problems if overused. For these reasons, Dr. Andrew Weil, a longtime advocate of flaxseed oil, now recommends hempseed oil to his patients.

DEFENDING YOUR LIFE

Your immune system is your key to preventing disease, fighting off illness, and living a long and healthy life. It is composed of white blood cells, and these white blood cells, along with all other proteins, are constructed with amino acids. Eight of these amino acids cannot be manufactured by the body, and must be supplied by our food; these are called the essential amino acids. Hempseed is one of the rare vegetable sources of all eight essential amino acids, and it is particularly rich in a rare one called edestin. Edestin is so important to the immune system that it has been studied for decades as a treatment for tuberculosis, cancer, and now AIDS.

SUPPLE SKIN

Hempseed oil is one of the few sources of gamma-linolenic acid (GLA), an EFA that resembles sebum, the natural lubricant in skin and hair. For this reason, personal hygiene products made with hempseed oil enhance the skin's softness and smoothness and help lend hair its natural sheen and body. GLA may also help treat psoriasis, eczema, dandruff, and other skin diseases.

A number of companies now have hempseed-based hair- and skin-care products on the market. These products include massage oil, lip balm, shampoo, conditioner, perfume, body soap, skin cream, facial scrub, and salve.

HEMP HUMMUS

With the protein-punch of hempseed, the EFAs of hempseed oil, the invigorating properties of garlic, and absolutely no THC, a bowl of this a day will keep the doctor, the DEA, and your less adventurous friends away.

    1 14-oz. can chickpeas, drained
        (reserve liquid)
    ¹/₄ cup liquid from chickpeas
    Juice of 1 lemon
    ¹/₂ cup ground roasted hempseed
    ¹/₂ cup pure hempseed oil
    4 garlic cloves
    ¹/₂ cup parsley

Mix all ingredients in blender or food processor until smooth. Add more chickpea liquid if needed. Serve as an appetizer (or main course, if garlic doesn't scare you!) with pita bread, bagel chips, or raw vegetables, and the world will indeed be a much improved place!

THE BREAKFAST
OF CHAMPIONS

Want to cut down on that morning coffee habit? Looking for a new brew for breakfast? Hempseed/coffee blends are now on the market, as well as a coffee-free beverage made with roasted hempseed and chicory. Roasted hempseeds eliminate some of the bitterness in coffee, cut down on the amount of caffeine, and provide an easy way of getting your essential fatty acids (EFAs). To get the complete hemp morning experience, brew with a reusable 100 percent hemp coffee filter.

HEMPEN ALE

There is one exception to the rule that you can't catch a buzz from industrial hemp. Hempen Ale, brewed by Frederick Brewing Company, of Frederick, Maryland, uses hempseed for 30 percent of its grain. According to Marjorie McGinnis, president of the brewery, "The hempseeds give it kind of a creamy head, and kind of an herbal, floral smell. It has kind of a nutty taste. It tastes like beer with a twist."

The chairman of Frederick Brewing Company, Kevin Brannon, says "We support those who are attempting to awaken policy makers to the vast potential of a renewed American hemp industry. We're doing our part—one beer at a time."

FEATHERED FRIENDS

Hempseed is the favorite food of birds everywhere. Four million pounds of it were sold for this purpose in the United States in 1937. Serious bird raisers have continued to import hempseed ever since. Birds fed hempseed get fewer diseases and live 20 percent longer than average. Chickens produce larger, oranger, more nutrient-rich eggs when hempseed is a part of their diet.

SEE? NO EVIL

Thousands of glaucoma sufferers have saved their vision by using cannabis. Glaucoma is a disease that prevents the fluid in the eyes from draining properly. This causes a buildup of inner ocular pressure, which when it gets too high can permanently damage the eyeball and even cause blindness. Smoking cannabis has proved to be the most effective way to relieve inner ocular pressure. It also avoids the damage to the liver and kidneys associated with traditional glaucoma medicines.

AIDS RELIEF

Two of the most debilitating symptoms of AIDS are nausea and lack of appetite. Cannabis alleviates both. By eliminating a patient's nausea and giving him "the munchies"—the famous side effect of smoking marijuana—the patient is able to take in nutrients badly needed to support the body's health.

THE CANCER ANSWER

Patients with cancer dread chemotherapy because it poisons the body and produces uncontrollable nausea. Many of these patients in the 1970s discovered that smoking marijuana instantly relieved their nausea and allowed them to lead more normal lives. Word spread, and soon medical studies revealed that marijuana was effective in more than 80 percent of cases. Nearly half the oncologists in the country have admitted that they would recommend marijuana to patients if the federal ban on the plant was lifted.

BREATHE EASY

Cannabis is a bronchodilator, meaning it expands the air passages and allows them to take in more fresh air. Because of this, it has been used to treat asthma for over 3,000 years. The relaxing effect of cannabis can also be helpful for someone suffering from an asthma attack.

AN ANTIBIOTIC

Cannabis juice has been used as a poultice to treat infections and wounds for centuries, and recent studies have revived interest in the plant's antibiotic properties. The natural juice makes an excellent disinfectant for ear or throat infections, and cannabis extract proved effective against oral herpes, gingivitis, and certain strains of staphylococci. THC killed herpes virus cells in a 1990 study at the University of South Florida, but so far the majority of the evidence for cannabis's antibacterial effects comes from folk wisdom rather than the laboratory.

AN IMMUNOSUPPRESSANT

Cannabis mildly suppresses the immune system, which appears to be just enough to take the edge off autoimmune diseases such as rheumatoid arthritis, colitis, Crohn's disease, and multiple sclerosis. These diseases are caused when the body's immune system mistakenly attacks its own cells, causing inflammation, pain, and poor functioning. Such chronic diseases are very difficult to treat and most often are barraged with steroids. The symptoms, however, can frequently be controlled with cannabis.

AN ANTICONVULSANT

Cannabis is extremely effective in relieving the spasms associated with epilepsy, muscular dystrophy, multiple sclerosis, and other convulsant diseases. Often it is able to prevent attacks entirely. Interestingly, though THC is somewhat effective in relieving spasms, the compound that has been found to be most effective is cannabidiol (CBD). CBD is found in much greater concentrations in industrial hemp than in medical marijuana, meaning that this drug could be legalized without legalizing psychoactive cannabis.

AN ANTI-INFLAMMATORY

The miraculous healing powers of cannabis apply to inflammation as well. Cannabis is more effective than aspirin or even hydrocortisone, and is the perfect choice for those with pruritus, dermatitis, edema, and other inflammatory diseases who do not want to submit their bodies to the ravages of steroids.

NO PAIN

Cannabis was the most popular remedy for migraines in the nineteenth century, and thousands still use it for just that purpose. As an analgesic its use goes back thousands of years. One of its most promising areas of modern use is in combination with morphine. A low dose of THC increases morphine's effect by 500 percent. This would allow doctors to use much less of this toxic drug to achieve the same level of pain relief.

Cannabis's power in relieving arthritic pain has been discovered by a growing number of elderly users in recent years. And if any group can strike fear into politicians' hearts and get medical marijuana legalized, it is the AARP.

THE IND PROGRAM

Did you know that the U.S. government supplies marijuana to eight people free of charge? The Investigative New Drug Program was started in 1975 to supply people suffering from glaucoma, cancer, and other incurable diseases with the only medicine that could help them—cannabis. The government grows its marijuana at the University of Mississippi, and between 1976 and 1990 supplied over 160,000 joints to needy patients.

The program was a huge success—and that was the problem. The contradiction of the government preaching "Just say no!" while supplying cannabis to grateful patients eventually received too much attention and the program closed to new patients in 1992. Still, the continuation of the program for eight remaining patients gives us all hope that the government will take a tip from itself and come to its senses.

MEDICINE FOR THE MASSES

Cannabis grows easily in almost every climate. This, combined with its wide range of healing applications, makes it ideal as a medicine for the home. It is virtually impossible to overdose on cannabis (cannabis is 40,000 times safer than aspirin in this regard), so a doctor's supervision is unnecessary. Cannabis helps take healing out of the hospital and put it back in the hands of citizens. In the future every family may keep a few hemp plants in the herb garden for instant self-medication.

MEDICINE FOR PENNIES

Cannabis, a natural plant, cannot be patented by any pharmaceutical company. Since they can't make any money from the plant, these companies have no interest in pursuing the research necessary to get FDA approval. They prefer to sell their lab-created chemical cures, a multibillion dollar industry.

A marijuana joint, meanwhile, sells for a few dollars and is more effective than many patented medicines. If it weren't for prohibition the price would probably be under a dollar. Cannabis could save the world's citizens trillions of dollars in health-care costs. Don't be surprised if one of the groups to embrace medical marijuana is the insurance industry, just as it has done with alternative health care, another money-saver.

JUST ASK JAMA

The *Journal of the American Medical Association* ran a commentary by Lester Grinspoon, M.D., and James Bakalar, J.D., stating:

"One of marijuana's greatest advantages as a medicine is its remarkable safety. It has little effect on major physiological functions. There is no known case of a lethal overdose. . . . Marijuana is also far less addictive and far less subject to abuse than many drugs now used as muscle relaxants, hypnotics, and analgesics. . . . The ostensible indifference of physicians should no longer be used as a justification for keeping this medicine in the shadows."

HOW ABOUT NEJM?

The *New England Journal of Medicine* is equally strong in its support of cannabis:

"A federal policy that prohibits physicians from alleviating suffering by prescribing marijuana for seriously ill patients is misguided, heavy-handed, and inhumane. . . . Whatever their reasons, federal officials are out of step with the public. . . . The government should change marijuana's status from that of a Schedule 1 drug (considered to be potentially addictive and with no current medical use) to that of a Schedule 2 drug (potentially addictive but with some accepted medical use) and regulate it accordingly. . . . Some physicians will have the courage to challenge the continued proscription of marijuana for the sick. Eventually, their actions will force the courts to adjudicate between the rights of those at death's door and the absolute power of bureaucrats whose decisions are based more on reflexive ideology and political correctness than on compassion."

CONSUMER REPORTS

A third ringing endorsement for medical marijuana came in May 1997 from a completely unexpected place: *Consumer Reports,* those watchdogs of quality.

"Since an unknown but probably substantial number of people are smoking marijuana with the expectation that it will help make their AIDS or terminal cancer more tolerable, *Consumer Reports* urges the Federal Government to permit further research in this area—to better determine the drug's efficacy and side effects.

"In the meantime, *Consumer Reports* believes that, for patients with advanced AIDS and terminal cancer, the apparent benefits some derive from smoking marijuana outweigh any substantiated or even suspected risks. In the same spirit the FDA uses to hasten the approval of cancer drugs, Federal laws should be relaxed in favor of states' rights to allow physicians to administer marijuana to their patients on a caring and compassionate basis."

THE BIG CURE?

The most miraculous medical application of cannabis may be yet to come. Studies have shown that THC reduces tumors in mice as much as 82 percent. Little research has been done in this area, but scientists are encouraged to get started anytime they want!

IT SAVED
STEPHEN JAY GOULD

Without marijuana one of our greatest scientists, Stephen Jay Gould, might not still be with us. Treated for the previously incurable cancer abdominal mesothelioma, his chemotherapy left him with incredible nausea that almost finished him. Reluctantly, he tried marijuana:

"Marijuana worked like a charm. . . . The sheer bliss of not experiencing nausea . . . was the greatest boost I received in all my years of treatment, and surely had a most important effect on my eventual cure. It is beyond my comprehension—and I fancy I am able to comprehend a lot, including much nonsense—that any humane person would withhold such a beneficial substance from people in such great need simply because others use it for different purposes."

SMOKED MEDICINE

A consistent argument from the National Institute of Health for why marijuana will never make good medicine is because it is smoked, and there are no other examples of a medicine that is smoked. Never mind the blatant tautology in this statement, the fact is that one of the reasons marijuana is such a good medicine is *because* it is smoked. Marinol, the government's own THC pill, has proved disastrously ineffective for treating chemotherapy because—surprise!—nauseous patients can't get the pill down. The beauty of marijuana's effect is that you can't vomit the smoke back up. Smoked medicine is a life saver. It is also many times less expensive than Marinol.

PSYCHOTHERAPY

Marijuana is frequently used by psychotherapists to treat depression—though this use is almost never reported. The few studies that have been done show mixed results—marijuana seems to increase patients' depression as often as it lifts it—but a number of people have been helped by marijuana's tendency to cause laughter and to give one a new perspective on one's problems.

Another psychotherapeutic quality of marijuana is its ability to reduce tension and anxiety. This can prove useful to create the relaxed, safe, trusting environment necessary for good therapy.

ALCOHOL THERAPY

As any substance abuse counselor can tell you, the percentage of alcoholics who ever successfully cure themselves through Alcoholics Anonymous or other programs is depressingly low. Something powerful needs to come into alcoholics lives to replace the booze that numbed their depression, and often there is nothing there.

A growing number of counselors are finding that marijuana is the ideal stepping stone to a drug-free lifestyle. Marijuana provides a cleaner and safer feeling of ecstasy than alcoholics had previously received from booze, and once the alcohol dependency is broken, marijuana proves far easier to give up because it isn't physically addictive.

HOMEOPATHY

More and more people are curing illnesses by turning away from invasive allopathic medicine and embracing gentle homeopathy. Homeopathy was as important a type of medicine as allopathy in the nineteenth century, but then the better financed allopathic community was able to wage a campaign against homeopathy, until allopathy became accepted as the only "real" medicine.

Times are changing, and many have rediscovered just how effective homeopathy can be, as well as cheaper and much less frightening. The juice of cannabis, made into a tincture, was one of the original and most popular homeopathic remedies, and could be used as such again. Doctors' reports indicate that it was useful in treating everything from earaches and tinnitus to muscle cramps, eye pain, and sexual problems. It seems to be particularly effective in treating nervous conditions of all kinds.

TRADITIONAL CHINESE MEDICINE

Cannabis's oldest medicinal use is in China, where it has been considered one of the "superior elixirs of immortality" for well over 3,000 years. The tops of female hemp plants are used to treat gout, malaria, rheumatism, and menstrual problems. Hempseed is eaten to retain fertility and strength, and to treat digestion and urinary difficulties. Crushed seeds are used on the skin to assuage abscesses, boils, pimples, and inflammation.

YOUR SHIVA CONNECTION

The Hindu pantheon is presided over by Shiva, the god of creation, destruction, and bliss. Shiva's affinity for cannabis is so well known that he is commonly called "Lord of Bhang" (bhang is a drink made of cannabis leaves). Hindus believe that to smoke cannabis is to commune with Shiva, to draw close to the joy of creation. And who's to say they're wrong?

SADDHUS

Judging from India, if you're going to be an ascetic, cannabis seems to make life a whole lot easier. India's ascetics—fervent devotees of the cult of Shiva known as saddhus—wander the countryside naked or in rags, living off handouts and owning nothing. They believe that this austere existence allows them to escape the soul-deadening effects of the material world, and they live in constant awareness of their divine inner natures. Smoking cannabis allows them to endure their constant physical discomfort and hunger, and to perceive Shiva in all his manifestations.

TANTRA

The Buddhist sect known as Tantra, currently gaining popularity in the West, has for millennia practiced religious rites in which cannabis played a key role. Tantra advocates embrace sensual activities such as eating and sex as a way of freeing yourself from your conscious mind and realizing your oneness with all of creation. Tantric practitioners generally begin by smoking or imbibing cannabis. This allows them to immerse themselves in the experiences to come and thus achieve higher states of spirituality.

AN APHRODISIAC

The reports are all anecdotal, of course. No official studies have been done. And far be it from me to suggest that it is possible to improve on the mind-blowing sex you have every day. But the persistent rumor has existed for centuries, so I'll just throw it out there: cannabis just may make sex even better. The increased sensitivity, the relaxing effect, and the general sense of well-being that it imparts could all contribute to this. And the world certainly needs more good sex. But don't take my word for it—find out for yourself.

RASTAFARIANISM

The heart and soul of the Rastafarian religion is their use of ganga. Characteristic qualities of cannabis use pervade all spiritual and sociological aspects of Rastafarianism: emphasis on inner truths and the cultivation of wisdom, daily meditation, a strong sense of community, tolerance of others, and a love of music and other pleasures. Ganga also forms a direct link to Rastafarianism's roots in the spiritual traditions of Africa, which used cannabis in identical ways.

RELIGIOUS FREEDOM

The Ethiopian Zion Coptic Church traces its use of cannabis in religious practices back more than 2,000 years. Though originally persecuted by the U.S. government for its use of cannabis as a holy sacrament, the church fought in court for its right to use a plant that was a traditional part of its religion and won. This has opened the door for others whose religious rights have been similarly quashed, such as the Navajo Nation, which recently was allowed to use peyote in its religious ceremonies.

MAKING BEAUTIFUL
MUSIC TOGETHER

Marijuana first gained popularity among jazz musicians in New Orleans early in this century. Was it coincidental that use of marijuana and the explosion of jazz creativity went hand in hand? Or did the plant help unlock a soulful and brilliant part of the American spirit? In any case, the association of marijuana with jazz musicians was so strong that Harry Anslinger, director of the Federal Bureau of Narcotics, once planned on busting Louis Armstrong, Count Basie, Duke Ellington, Gene Krupa, Cab Calloway, Jimmy Dorsey, and Dizzy Gillespie, among others. Fortunately, his supervisor thought better of his plans.

VOILA, CIVILIZATION!

The oldest evidence of cannabis use places it back in India and China some 10,000 years ago. This is also when the first civilizations arose. Coincidence? Some don't think so.

"It would be wryly interesting," Carl Sagan observed in *The Dragons of Eden,* "if in human history the cultivation of marijuana led generally to the invention of agriculture, and thereby to civilization."

Philosopher Terence McKenna takes this idea a step further. He believes that cannabis and other psychotropic plants gave our neanderthal consciousness a swift kick in the neurons, sparking insights that heralded the birth of modern man.

THE GREAT NEGOTIATOR

Cannabis is famous for getting people to find common ground, but this ability was taken to new heights in nineteenth-century Africa. A chieftain whose tribe had recently conquered many other tribes in the Belgian Congo was having trouble getting his new subjects, who each had their own religion, to stop warring with each other. He destroyed their religious icons and instead supplied them with cannabis. They quickly saw the error in their ways and, far from harboring ill will toward one another, united under the name "sons of cannabis."

THE WAR CURE

Marijuana's role in ending the Vietnam war should not be downplayed. There is no telling how many lives it helped to save. Its uncanny knack for bringing feelings of peacefulness, and for helping users to recognize their fellowship with all other beings on the planet, is to blame. In Vietnam, many soldiers were introduced to marijuana for the first time. Suddenly smoking a joint and enjoying the day seemed like a much better way to kill time than slogging through mud and jungles. It certainly made more sense than killing *people* you didn't even know.

On the homefront, marijuana helped many young people to feel a kinship with the "enemy," and to see through the belligerent policies of the government. Public sentiment turned against the war, and the country was changed forever.

TURNING ON, TUNING OUT

Cannabis has long been a thorn in the side of social institutions that want to keep people from thinking too hard by keeping them working too hard. This occurred with the Sufis in fourteenth-century Islam, who favored direct, ecstatic communion with the divine over the repressive rules of orthodox Islamism; the blissful Shaivites in India under British rule; and most famously with the hippy generation in the United States in the 1960s.

Capable of creating an environment conducive to creative thinking, and supremely affordable, marijuana allowed a massive change of consciousness to occur in the 1960s. It did not *create* this change of consciousness, it just loosened the pressure to conform that had been dominant and allowed a natural evolution to take place.

An eternal enemy of totalitarianism, repression, and agression, the plant has probably saved societies and civilizations from themselves more times than anyone will ever know.

IT'S FUNNY

During the campaign for Proposition 215 in California, Gary Trudeau made the proposition the focus of a hilarious series of *Doonesbury* cartoons mocking Dan Lungren, the Attorney General of California. True to form, Lungren attempted to have the cartoons censored in the California papers. Not only were they not censored, but the negative publicity Lungren received for his actions helped to turn the campaign around.

IT'S A
STEPPING-STONE DRUG

To greater medical rights, that is. Propositions 215 in California and 200 in Arizona, and the totalitarian tactics state and federal governments used to try and suppress these measures, have awakened the American public to the realization that they should have much greater medical rights than they do. The success of Californians for Medical Rights, the group that fought for Proposition 215, has led to the founding of Americans for Medical Rights, which campaigns for medical marijuana across the country. Exposure to this issue has brought an influx of contributions to other groups campaigning for the clinical and therapeutic use of other psychedelics such as LSD and MDMA.

THE DRUG OF CHOICE (1)

Every culture has its drug of choice. For modern civilization, it's alcohol. Alcohol provides a foggy buzz, but along with it come some less desirable characteristics. On the mild side, it is a huge source of empty calories, fattening us up but nutritionally barren. More seriously, alcoholism kills over 100,000 people a year and ruins the lives of many more. Cirrhosis of the liver and other diseases add to alcohol's deadly toll.

In contrast, marijuana is nonaddictive and is not linked to any health conditions. It is a remark- ably safe drug that would save lives as well as the huge health-care costs associated with alcohol. It should be our drug of choice for the coming millennium.

THE DRUG OF CHOICE (2)

The advantage of marijuana being as simple a thing as a dried plant is often overlooked. This makes it the ideal drug of choice from a conservation standpoint. Producing alcohol requires harvesting huge quantities of grain with gas-powered machinery, trucking that grain to breweries and distilleries, steeping it in vats of clean water, boiling it for hours, creating glass bottles to store it, and finally trucking the cumbersome stuff to market. Marijuana, on the other hand, is incredibly light on the environment. Grown locally in almost all areas of the country, harvested in small amounts by hand, dried naturally, and sold directly, it uses no energy, requires no factories or infrastructure, and creates no waste. It is an exemplary industry.

WAR ON DRUGS

"There never was a good war or a bad peace," said Benjamin Franklin. Perhaps the Drug Czar should listen to him. More than $30 billion a year is spent on the War on Drugs, a war that has achieved nothing but suffering for untold numbers of people. Thousands have had their lives ruined, many have been killed. And when you begin to think of the incredible good that might have been done with $30 billion a year, you realize it is a very bad war.

Marijuana is far and away the most benign drug included in the War on Drugs, and should be part of an immediate armistice.

THE GREAT
AMERICAN WAY

"Why, boys, when I was seventeen I walked into the jungle, and when I was twenty-one I walked out. And by God I was rich."

Arthur Miller's famous line from *Death of a Salesman* sums up the great American dream, and marijuana growers throughout the country are making this dream happen with hard work, green thumbs, and personal risk. The government estimates that the marijuana industry grosses over $50 billion a year and employs more than one million people, making it one of the most profitable industries in the country.

The problem? It's all tax free. Obviously, nobody's marijuana income shows up on their W-2s. This amounts to $5 billion in lost revenue for the United States. Can we afford to keep this plant illegal anymore?

THE PRISON BOOM

The United States is building prisons like there is no tomorrow, and for a growing number of young people in this country there may not be. The U.S. prison population has doubled in the last fifteen years, almost entirely because of the surging number of drug offenders. More than $5 billion was spent on new prisons in 1995, and this number continues to rise. Equally staggering is the fact that a full 10 percent of law enforcement budgets nationwide goes to busting marijuana users. Add to this the $20,000 that it costs to keep each inmate in jail for one year and you realize just how much the War on Drugs is costing us. Let's pocket the $5 billion and stop sending marijuana users to jail.

EXCISE TAXES

The highest revenues we are gypping ourselves out of by keeping marijuana illegal come from excise taxes. Tobacco cigarettes currently sell for about 10 cents a piece, and since marijuana production costs are similar, joints could be sold for the same price with profit margins equivalent to those of tobacco companies. Since nobody wants marijuana to be that inexpensive, however, huge excise taxes could be placed on it, higher than those on cigarettes or alcohol, and it would still be profitable. A tax of $1.90 per joint would raise the price to $2, similar to half a six-pack of beer or half a bottle of wine, either of which produces similar levels of intoxication to one joint. An estimated 20 million joints are smoked in the United States each day, so this $1.90 excise tax would generate $13.9 billion a year.

THE BOTTOM LINE

How much total revenue would a regulated marijuana industry generate for the United States? The
answer is shocking.

Law enforcement budget for marijuana interdiction	$ 5	billion
Cost of new prisons to house marijuana criminals	$ 5	billion
Lost income tax	$ 5	billion
Excise taxes	$13.9	billion
Sales tax (@ 5%)	$ 2.5	billion
TOTAL ANNUAL REVENUES	$31.4	billion

Can our nation afford to maintain this fool-
hardy stance on cannabis?

SOFT ON CRIME

The biggest supporter of crime in America is Drug Czar General Barry McCaffrey. His endorsement of mandatory minimum sentences for drug offenders has done more to put criminals on the streets than organized crime ever has. Why? Because our prison system, which is perfectly adequate to house all other criminals, cannot handle the flood of drug offenders being sent to it.

In 1970 just 16 percent of federal prison inmates were drug offenders. By 1996 this number was 61 percent. What happened to all the violent criminals? They've been set free, of course, to make room for the marijuana smokers.

Since the mandatory minimum drug bill in 1986, the average time served for violent crimes has *declined* by a third, while the average time served for drug violations has risen proportionately. Remember this: every marijuana user sent to jail means the release of a hardened criminal. Does the Drug Czar make you feel safer now?

THE MONSTER FACTORY

Half a million marijuana users are arrested each year, mostly young people. For many it is their first brush with the law. Most of these people would never think of harming another human being, yet because of mandatory minimum sentences they are forced into the prison system, where they are physically attacked, raped, exposed to the most vile behavior imaginable, and inculcated into the ways of crime by convicts with far more experience than them. By the time they are released—making way for the next influx of innocents—they are dangerous criminals indeed.

You see, the entire prison system is a highly successful (and free) university of crime, with young people taught what they need to know to commit crimes and then sent back to the world to ply their trade. The ones with a real knack for it generally return to prison for postgraduate studies.

DANGEROUS IMPORTS

Half of the marijuana consumed in the United States is imported. Besides contributing significantly to our trade imbalance, this presents many dangers to consumers and to our entire agricultural system. Marijuana is far and away the largest crop that is brought into the United States without being inspected. Since the crop is also grown and processed without any official supervision, it is wide open to contamination. Marijuana shipments captured at the border have been found to contain illegal herbicides, dangerous molds, insect bodies and eggs, even animal feces.

Most urgently, the chance of this uninspected crop bringing in new insect pests that cause widespread crop damage is extremely worrisome. One only has to remember the Mediterranean fruit fly disaster of the 1980s to realize the harm this could cause.

The only solution, of course, is to have a legal, domestic, regulated marijuana industry.

POISONING THE PEOPLE

In a classic example of cutting off their nose to spite their face, the Reagan administration had the bright idea of spraying our national forests with paraquat, a deadly herbicide. The idea was that this was where some marijuana was being grown, so it would kill the plants, along with everything else in the vicinity, and would poison anyone who consumed the illegal substance. Paraquat causes lung lesions, intestinal disorders, convulsions, kidney damage, respiratory failure, and, ultimately, death. Despite objections from local health officials that "the death penalty for marijuana is too severe," the spraying went on. Just another way that your government is out there protecting you.

DUTCH TREAT

In 1976 the Netherlands began a policy of tolerating possession of up to one ounce of cannabis. Soon "coffee shops" sprung up throughout the nation selling a variety of strains of cannabis and hashish. The result? Massive crime and a stampede of children toward drug addiction? Hardly.

A mere 3 percent of Dutch teenagers use cannabis, a far cry from the U.S. rate. Once the "outlaw" attraction was gone, most teens lost interest in cannabis. Dutch prisons also don't suffer from the overcrowding problems common in the United States. This de facto legalization has allowed the Netherlands to concentrate on treatment, rather than incarceration, for users of hard drugs such as cocaine and heroin, which has saved countless lives.

The Dutch stance on cannabis has generated thousands of jobs, millions of dollars, and worldwide praise and goodwill. Naturally, this progressive country is also reaping the rewards of being Europe's leader in industrial hemp production and technology.

BUDDING PROSPECTS

Cannabis makes great fiction. Check out *The Thousand and One Nights,* in which hashish figures in several tales, or Rabelais's bawdy satire *Gargantua and Pantagruel.* Check out James Allen's 1900 novel *The Reign of Law: A Tale of the Kentucky Hemp Fields,* Guy Mount's *The Marijuana Mystery,* and Rand Clifford's *Castling.* Best of all, check out T. Coraghessen Boyle's novel *Budding Prospects,* a hilarious account of hapless marijuana growers in the mountains of Northern California.

PAPER TRADE

The subject of hemp is supporting a small but growing number of dedicated researchers, activists, and journalists who are turning out some excellent books and journals. Some of the information in this book came from the following sources. I urge those who want to deepen their knowledge on this subject to read them:

The Emperor Wears No Clothes, by Jack Herer
The Great Book of Hemp, by Rowan Robinson
Hemp for Health, by Chris Conrad
Hemp: Lifeline to the Future, by Chris Conrad
Hempworld Magazine, edited by Mari Kane
Why Marijuana Should Be Legal, by Ed Rosenthal
    and Steve Kubby

?

You tell us. Have you thought of another way that hemp can help to save the world? Park Street Press and I would love to hear from you. Visit the web site at www.gotoit.com or send us e-mail at hemp@gotoit.com. Together we can make a difference!